The Couch Potato's Guide To Getting Fit

Weight Loss, Strength Training & Physical Rehabilitation with the Power of Thought

I0440174

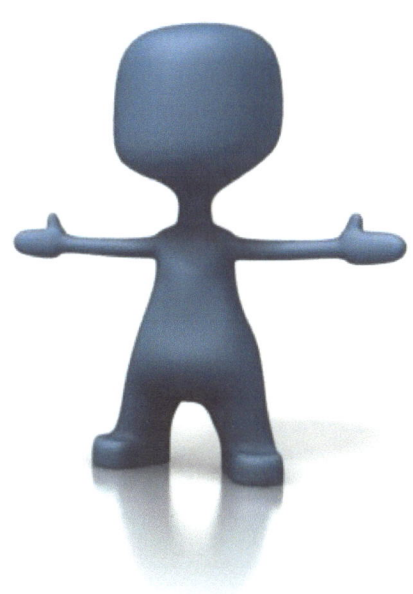

By: Patrick Sean Cook

The Couch Potato's Guide To Getting Fit

The Couch Potato's Guide To Getting Fit

Table of Contents

Chapter 1 - Mental Fitness

"Whenever I feel the need to exercise, I lie down until it goes away."

- Robert Maynard Hutchins

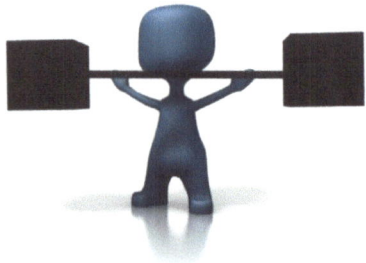

My stationary friends, the single greatest challenge facing the couch potato community today, is that of physical fitness, or lack thereof.

There are literally thousands of weight loss and exercise programs available, but if any of them had actually worked, you would not likely be reading this book.

I have climbed the mountain, stared into the angry eye of the abyss, snatched the pebble from its metaphorical hand, and brought back the answers to the questions that no one asked me to find.

1. Is it possible to lose body fat without dietary or caloric restrictions?

2. Is it possible to increase muscle mass and strength without physically moving?

Heady questions indeed, stupid, but heady. Throwing caution to the wind, I dredged into the depths few have dared to go. Into the world of the tedious and the tiresome, the mind deadening masses of over stuffed words that is scientific documentation. On and on I searched. I began to wonder if perhaps my search was in vain.

And then I found it!

I'm about to drop a double-knee face-breaker of knowledge. A wheel-kicking palm strike of vicious intellectual profoundness. A cross-chopping forearm shiver of life changing wisdom.

Scientific studies over the past decade prove, you can in fact lose body fat, and gain muscle mass and strength, using only the power of your thoughts!

Sitting perfectly still, you can grow strong lean muscle, and lose body fat, without any physical movement what so ever.

Mic dropped...

I'm not talking about minor changes in the body, go big or go home son! I'm talking about results that are comparable to actual physical exercise, and in some cases, exceed the positive effects of traditional physical exercise.

Results from imagined exercise, counter to what you'd expect, actually last longer than those gained from traditional physical exercise. Shut up, are you serious? I will not shut up, and I'm totally being serious.

Even more astounding, repeated thought exercise has been found effective in preventing Alzheimer's disease and cognitive decline, building physically stronger neuromuscular pathways in the brain.

Our biggest weakness, just sitting around and doing nothing, will become our greatest strength. Thought exercise actually encourages a person to perform them while in a resting position. We have already mastered this art form. We have been trailblazers in the field of physical fitness without even knowing it.

Why this works:

Brain imaging scans show that thought exercise activates the same portions of the brain as physical exercise.

In other words, your brain does not know the difference between thought exercise and physical exercise. Per Kai Miller, Physicist Stanford University.

Read that again, and let it sink in.

We have found a flaw in the system that we can exploit to our benefit. Sure we could go out for a run, but why not just imagine ourselves going for a run instead? Your brain won't know the difference, and as you'll see, positive physical results will ensue.

I give you the Couch Potato's Guide to Getting Fit.

Chapter 2 - The Scientific Stuff Begins

"I'm 99% sure no one would run marathons if they weren't allowed to talk about running marathons."

- Mike Vanatta

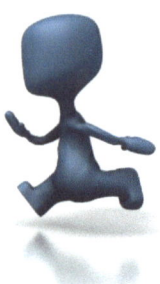

The following is in no way meant as a comprehensive list of available supportive cognitive studies, but a small sample to demonstrate the power of "mind over matter".

Now on with the science man!

Brian Clark, of Ohio University used twenty-nine volunteers to produce a study measuring wrist strength. All subjects experienced the joy of having their wrists wrapped in surgical casts for an entire month.

Half of these lucky recruits performed mental wrist exercises, for only eleven minutes per day, five days a week, sitting perfectly still, imagining that they were moving their immobilized wrists. Fun times to be sure.

When the casts were removed they found that those who had performed mental exercises had wrists that were two times stronger than those who did nothing at all.

Think about that, twice the physical strength without physical exercise. This stuff is sounding pretty good about now, let's keep going.

Clark also found that those who performed imaginary exercises had stronger neuromuscular pathways, while those of the mentally lazy volunteers had weaker pathways, that were beginning to degrade.

So mental exercise increases your physical brain's strength, while a lack of mental stimulation, has been proven detrimental to your brain's physical health.

Now imagine the benefits for those going through rehabilitation and recovery from injury. The use of imagined exercise would dramatically reduce recuperation time typically spent building back up weakened muscle groups, while at the same time increasing strength without risk of injury.

In a study that focused on the volunteers fingers, Guang Yue of the Cleveland Clinic, found that imaginary exercise increased the subjects finger strength by thirty-five percent.

Another of Yue's studies focused on the bicep muscle and found that volunteers who visualized bicep movement exercises showed an increase of bicep strength of 13.5 percent.

"That suggests you can increase muscle strength solely by sending a larger signal to the motor neurons from the brain." Dr. Yue.

Those who participated in Yue's studies were tested every two weeks, and it was found that they maintained their increased strength for three months after the mental training had stopped!

While the results from physical exercise begin to fade within the first two to four weeks after exercise stopped, per the research of Iñigo Mujika, Sabino Padilla and Tibor Hortobagyi.

The fact that mental exercise maintains strength two months longer than physical exercise should be blowing your mind right about now. Let's pick those brains off the floor, and shovel them back in, because we are not done yet.

From the book, The Brain That Changes Itself, psychiatrist and researcher Norman Doidge, MD, states that thoughts can literally alter brain anatomy by switching your genes on and off.

Can you believe that? Your thoughts, or lack there of, have a physical impact on your genetic makeup.

This is Jedi mind stuff we're talking about here, using the power of the force, our thoughts, to control matter.

"People who simply imagined doing strength-training exercises increased their muscle strength by 22 percent, compared to 30 percent among those who physically did the exercise." per Dr. Joseph Mercola.

Important to note, all the results found in this book were achieved by beginners to the process of imaginary exercise including those of Dr. Mercola.

As we know, thought exercise has been found to build actual physical neuro connections, which get stronger over time.

It is therefore highly likely that continued and repeated mental exercise over a longer duration of time, may produce results that even surpass those of physical exercise.

Chapter 3 - Thought Induced Weight Loss

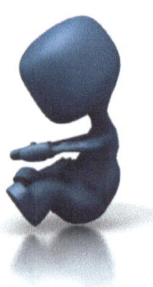

The dream is here y'all, no more counting calories or sacrificing what you love to eat. Let's take a trip to Harvard University.

Harvard researchers monitored two groups of hotel staff workers. One set of workers was told by the researchers that their daily work qualified as exercise, the other was not. Their bio-metrics were recorded and tracked throughout the study.

After four weeks, those who believed their work was a form of exercise had decreases in weight, blood pressure, body fat, waist-to-hip ratio, and body mass index, even though their behaviors and diet had not changed.

These people added no additional exercise, cut no calories, and still lost weight, body fat and had lower blood pressure. Starting to love me some science right about now, how about you?

We've been sold the idea, that to achieve weight loss results, one must sacrifice either to the caloric gods, or to the physical expenditure gods. But it seems a change in our perspective about exercise was just as powerful.

A simple suggestion by an authority figure resulted in positive physical changes in the human body, thereby shattering the myth of "no pain, no gain." I wonder what kind of results could have been achieved if mental exercise was incorporated into the study?

How do you suppose thought exercise could benefit the morbidly obese, who might be at risk of injury or be unable to safely perform physical exercise?

More on how Brain Exercise Prevents Cognitive Decline

The study, Preventing Alzheimer's Disease and Cognitive Decline, involved more than 2,800 adults 65 and older and found that when people kept their minds active, their thinking skills are less likely to decline.

Those who attended the mental training sessions, over a six week period, showed improvements in memory, reasoning, and speed of processing information.

Studies involving animals have shown that keeping the mind active reduces the amount of brain cell damage associated with Alzheimer's. It also supports the growth of new nerve cells, and prompts nerve cell messages to each other.

Stronger neuromuscular pathways are physically created during the process of mental exercise, which has been shown to stave off dementia, reduce memory loss, and increase processing of information. (William Blahd, MD, Aug 2014)

I think by now most would agree, that nursing homes across the globe, should start implementing mental exercise programs immediately.

Chapter 4 - The Establishment Psychosis

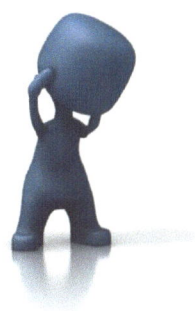

Well if mental exercise is so beneficial, why isn't it being done everywhere?

Establishments are resistant to change, as I'm sure you are well aware. The information provided in this book is but a small sample of what has been available to the clinical establishment for well over a decade.

The discoveries found in this book, have so far, fallen on deaf ears. It has happened before many times, much to the detriment of humanity.

One such case was in the mid 19th century, where it was common practice for medical students and professors at teaching hospitals to perform barehanded autopsies on women who had died the day before of "childbed fever".

These same doctors would then go on rounds to examine laboring women about to deliver. Not surprisingly, the mortality rates for the mother were 10 to 20 times higher when performed at a hospital, compared to those by a mid-wife. Good job Doc's.

Dr. Ignaz Semmelweis had the nerve to claim that it was the doctors themselves, that were putting patient's life at risk. Recommending both the washing of hands and that practicing obstetricians abstain from performing autopsies on women who had died of the fever, out of an obligation to society. What a psychopath.

This was of course met with rage and anger from his colleagues. How dare he accuse them of being the cause of the patients demise!

They rebutted that the problem of childbed fever could not be solved, because each patient was different, and therefore each cause of death was different, and thus could not be compared.

Besides, the prevailing theory was satisfactory, that the women had obviously died because their bodies, in that delicate state, could not stand the shock of male eyes upon their nakedness.

The discussion was to be closed and the Dr. Was to be shunned by his fellow doctors. Madness won the day, and ironically it was Dr. Semmelweis himself that was eventually committed to an insane asylum, where he promptly died two weeks later.

The practice of washing your hands was eventually accepted in Europe of course, but it took even longer before it became accepted in the United States.

It was still considered ridiculous, outrageous, and even threats of punishment against doctors who caved into such a frivolous suggestion.

We have always put far too much faith in those with power. We need to question more, and challenge outdated beliefs as they are found.

Blindly following what has always been, when evidence to the contrary is staring you right in the face, is a sure way to repeat the mistakes of the past.

Chapter 5 - How to Mentally Exercise

"I used to jog but the ice cubes kept falling out of my glass."

- David Lee Roth

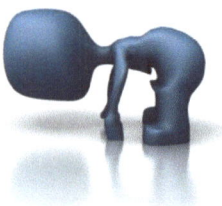

This is by far the easiest section of the book to follow. There are no special tricks or mental abilities required to succeed. And remember the more you practice, the stronger your mental and physical muscles will be.

Have your mind set on succeeding, your thoughts are strong and your body will respond.

One thing we do need to consider is from what perspective will you mentally view your virtual exercises from?

What I mean is when you close your eyes, do you see yourself in the first person or third person perspective?

1st person perspective - you visualize all your movement from the point of view of your imaginary eyes, just as you would during physical activity.

You have a limited view of your body. If you are doing a push-up for example, you likely can visualize your arms and hands as they press on the ground.

3rd person perspective - your view is from outside of your body, looking at it from above or from the side.

You have a clear image of your entire body and some of your surroundings as you complete each imaginary movement. Busting out rep after rep like a champ.

For myself, I like to switch between perspectives every so often to keep things interesting. I find the 1st person perspective of mental exercises more challenging for some reason.

It's probably just all in my head.

Decide on a location

Find a comfortable resting position. This could be literally anywhere but should be a place with limited distractions. The more focus you can apply to the task at hand, the better your results will be.

Anytime you are at rest is an opportunity to train. At your desk during a few minutes of down time, on the bus or subway on your way to work, or even when you are in the restroom.

Boring conversations are a great time for imaginary exercises. Drone on about the dry wall project my man, I'm doing virtual crunches.

Make it a habit

Mental exercise like anything gets easier the more you do it. Habits are formed when you do things over and over.

This is the most important step in the process. Find a way to incorporate mental training into your daily routine.

It is estimated that up to ninety percent of our daily behavior is habitual. We are creatures of habit, be they conscious or unconscious, healthy or unhealthy.

The greatest obstacle to positive habit forming is that it usually involves giving up an existing bad habit to be successful. Trying to replace smoking with chewing gum for example, not an equitable trade off most would agree.

The best thing about starting a mental exercise habit is the fact that you don't have to give up an existing bad habit in order to see positive results. Just add mental exercise to your list of current habits.

Beginners

For the first five days of training I recommend three short sessions, of no more than five minutes each spread throughout the day, morning, mid-day, and night.

By increasing the frequency of practice we can speed up the habit forming process.

Chapter 6 - The Program

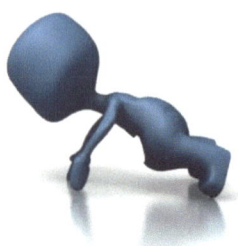

Like most successful physical exercise programs, I recommend that you incorporate a wide variety of diverse activities into your mental exercise program to prevent boredom.

I've started you off with three categories to select from: Aerobic, Strength Building, and Flexibility.

Your Goal should be 15 minutes of mental exercise each day, 5 days a week.

During your mental exercise, try to focus on the muscle groups that would physically be engaged as you perform each action.

If you are going on a mental run for instance, think of your legs and arms pumping and in constant motion, and that your core is engaged.

Change the mental location and conditions often. Why not take a run on the beach where you can imagine a more interesting landscape? The sand also could add additional mental resistance, because it's harder to run in sand than on concrete.

Or perhaps running uphill for even more of a challenge. Why not run up and over an entire mountain of sand while we are at it?

Tired of lifting virtual weights, why not mentally lift motorcycles or cars?

You might try some mental sports. How about an imagined basketball game against Micheal Jordan, and win?

A typical mental exercise session might include:

Aerobics for 5 minutes, Muscle Building for 5 minutes, Flexibility for 5 minutes = 15 minutes Total

Category 1 - Mental Aerobics

Running, Dancing, Jogging, Swimming, Biking, Tennis, Basketball, Mountain Climbing, Rowing, Jumping Rope

Category 2 - Mental Strength and Muscle Building

Bench Press - is performed while lying face up on a bench, by pushing a weight away from the chest.

Leg Press - The leg press is performed while seated by pushing a weight away from the body with the feet. It is a compound exercise that also involves the glutes and, to a lesser extent, the hamstrings and the calves.

Arm Curl - is performed while standing or seated, with hands hanging down holding weights (palms facing forwards), by curling them up to the shoulders.

Squat - The squat is performed by squatting down with a weight held across the upper back under neck and standing up straight again.

Deadlift - The deadlift is performed by squatting down and lifting a weight off the floor with the hand until standing up straight again.

Lunge - is performed by one leg is positioned forward with knee bent and foot flat on the ground while the other leg is positioned behind.

Pull-Up - is performed by hanging from a chin-up bar above head height with the palms facing forward and pulling the body up so the chin reaches or passes the bar.

Push-Up - performed in a prone position by raising and lowering the body using the arms.

Sit-Up - is performed lying with the back on the floor, typically with the arms across the chest or hands behind the head and the knees bent, raising your head to your knees. Sit-up have a fuller range of motion than crunches.

Crunch - is performed while lying face up on the floor with knees bent, by curling the shoulders up towards the pelvis

Leg Raise -is performed while sitting on a bench or flat on the floor by raising the knees towards the shoulders, or legs to a vertical upright position.

Category 3 - Mental Flexibility and Balance

Tia Chi, Pilates, Yoga, Stretching Legs, Arms, Back, Core, Standing On One Foot, Water Aerobics,

What other activities can you think of?

Chapter 7 - In the End

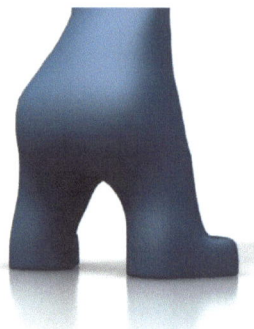

Visual exercise has been shown to increase physical muscles and maintain strength over a longer duration when compared to physical exercise.

Weight loss, lower blood pressure, lower body fat, lower waist-to-hip ratio, and lower body mass index were all accomplished with the power of thought alone.

Daily mental exercise also prevents cognitive decline and cognitive disease improving the quality of life.

Some applications for mental exercise include: nursing homes, hospitals, sports medicine, rehabilitation and recovery to name a few.

A mental exercise program could be implemented virtually anywhere with no additional expenditures. It is also clear that imaginary exercise could also play an important role in terms of reducing overall health care costs through preventive care.

I hope you come away from this book with a new appreciation and perspective on the power thought.

Visual exercise is appropriate, safe and effective for the entire spectrum of fitness levels, from professional athlete to couch potato.

Shout it from the rooftops, talk to your doctors, talk to your friends, call them from your couch, but get the message out about the importance of mental exercise.

It costs nothing but a few minutes of your time, and will substantially improve your quality of life as you get older.

We live in a world of distractions, with everyone and everything constantly fighting for our attention. It is more important than ever to take a break from your busy life, to find a quiet place, and think.

"The day science begins to study nonphysical phenomena, it will make more progress in one decade than in all previous centuries of its existence."

- Nikola Tesla

References

How to Grow Stronger Without Lifting Weights - Scientific America, by Clayton Mosher, Dec 2014 (Brian Clark, Guang Yue, Kai Miller)

http://www.scientificamerican.com/article/how-to-grow-stronger-without-lifting-weights/

How You Can Easily Exercise Without ANY Equipment, or Even Working Out - Joseph Mercola, Feb 2013

http://fitness.mercola.com/sites/fitness/archive/2013/02/08/simple-activity-increases-muscle-strength.aspx

How Quickly Do You Lose Gains from Strength Training? And, Could Taking a Break Actually Benefit You? - Runners Connect, John Davis

https://runnersconnect.net/running-training-articles/how-does-a-break-from-strength-training-impact-running-performance-a-look-at-the-scientific-research/

Thinking about exercise 'can beef up biceps' - The Telegraph, Robert Uhlig, Nov 2001 (Guang Yue)

http://www.telegraph.co.uk/news/worldnews/northamerica/usa/1363146/Thinking-about-exercise-can-beef-up-biceps.html

Brain Exercises and Dementia - WebMD, William Blahd, MD

http://www.webmd.com/alzheimers/guide/preventing-dementia-brain-exercises

In 1850, Ignaz Semmelweis saved lives with three words: wash your hands - PBS, Dr. Howard Markel, May 2015

http://www.pbs.org/newshour/updates/ignaz-semmelweis-doctor-prescribed-hand-washing/

Preventing Alzheimer's Disease and Cognitive Decline,Evidence Reports/Technology Assessments No. 193, John W Williams, MD, MPH, Brenda L Plassman, PhD, James Burke, MD, PhD,Tracey Holsinger, MD, and Sophiya Benjamin, MD. April 2010

http://www.ncbi.nlm.nih.gov/books/NBK47456/

Character "Blu" created by macouno. Released under Creative Commons Attribution 3.0.

Images created in Blender by Patrick Sean Cook

www.ingramcontent.com/pod-product-compliance
Lightning Source LLC
Chambersburg PA
CBHW050921290526
45792CB00002B/838